K.I.S.S.

Keeping It Sanely Simple

A Breast Cancer Guide

K.I.S.S.

Keeping It Sanely Simple

A Breast Cancer Guide

(The "Stuff" Nobody Tells You)

Stacey W. Dimmer, M.S.
Survivor

**K.I.S.S. is not intended to take the place
of medical advice by your physicians. It is
designed as a guide to help you through the journey.**

ISBN 978-0-557-48987-9

In Honor of Women Who:

Have,

Are,

And Will

Dedicated to Pete, My Hero

In Memory of DJP.

It Was an Honor.

Foreward

I must confess that this is my first endeavor in a long time writing something other than notes and orders in patients' charts. It was very kind of Stacey to ask me to compose this foreward, considering all of the trials and tribulations she suffered due to my efforts (although, admittedly, they were done on her behalf)! But that, so often, is the case in our line of work; patients often get hurt, in small ways and big, while being helped. The problems encountered on this journey run the gamut from the minor, albeit irritating, logistical ones to the sometimes severe and life-threatening physical ones. Despite their best efforts, there are so many issues that a nurse or a physician doesn't cover with a patient who is undergoing cancer treatment. Personally, I discovered a lot while reading this book. It was quite an eye-opener to read about the problems that Stacey addresses and to realize that, boy, I didn't even think that was an issue.

Stacey is well-suited to write this book—not only does she have a medical background, but she went through the whole range of treatments for her breast cancer. She also experienced the whole spectrum of side effects—including some rare and unusual ones. Being blessed with a way with words, she has been able to do justice to her objective of utilizing her background and experiences to help and guide others.

Advice is most helpful when served up in small and easy-to-digest packages. This is what this book is able to achieve. I would like to make special mention of the section on postsurgical care. I would never have known how to deal with many of the problems, even if I had thought about them (case in point: the best type of clothing to wear after a mastectomy). Someone with a patient's perspective is best suited to share this information, and this book truly illustrates that.

It can be difficult for someone to relive their experiences of surgery and chemotherapy, and to revisit their fears and apprehensions—which Stacey would have had to do to write this book. Having closely witnessed her determination, her humor, and her knowledge of her condition, I am not surprised that she has been able to do so. Indeed, the book reflects many of those qualities. It has helped me broaden my vision and hopefully will improve my ability to take care of my patients—a bigger task than just treating them. I am confident that this book will be a great guide and valuable resource to patients and their families.

Anup Lal, M.D.
Blue Water Oncology

Acknowledgements

My appreciation to my nephew, Marco Eadie. Thanks, Kiddo!

Thanks to R.J. King, editor, *DBusiness* magazine, for sharing his expertise.

Jane-Bob and Bug, you sent so much love during the dark days.

Vickie, E., Bren-doon, Scottie, and Jen, thank you for your help with anything and everything "computer".

Michelle, you give "sanity" a new meaning.

And, most of all, thanks to my husband for his continued unconditional love.

"A Quick Look"

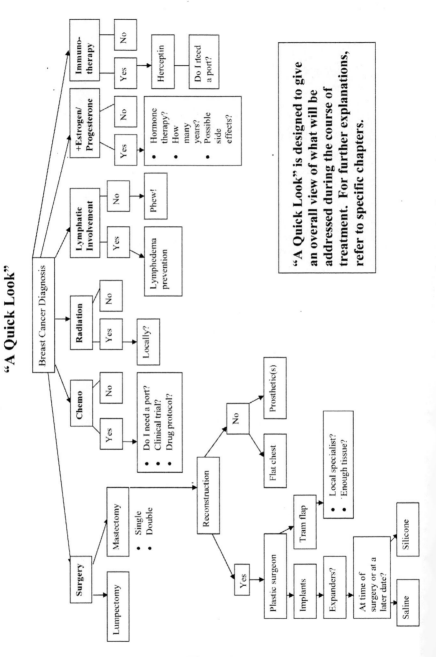

Figure 1

Index

INTRODUCTION

Introduction

Breast Cancer…keeping it simple...really?

When you're told you have breast cancer, you feel like you're a deer caught in the headlights. Big words that mean nothing to you are being hurled your way, decisions need to be made, and you're still trying to comprehend what was just said...huh?...no, that can't be right.

K.I.S.S. is about what "nobody" tells you after you've been diagnosed with breast cancer. This book provides easy-to-access information that's designed to help you get through the "day-to-day" issues...kind of like Heloise's helpful hints for the breast cancer patient. A woman may have up to a five-year journey (yes, really) of "dancing with the devil," and that doesn't include follow-up care. Each section provides easy-to-understand and helpful information in bullet-style reading. Information doesn't have to be complicated to be useful.

Generally, upon diagnosis the patient is handed reading materials about cancer that are more like science books; you need a Ph.D. to weed through them. When I was handed a two-inch-thick book, my first thought was, "Are they nuts?" That wasn't a good sign, since I'm a health care provider and have a master's degree in science. I wondered when I was ever going to read it, let alone understand what it all said. Honestly, at that moment I really couldn't care about the molecular structure of my cancer cells or the statistics pertaining to the incidence of breast cancer in the state of Rhode Island. I was so overwhelmed with the diagnosis itself, I wasn't even sure what questions I needed to ask the doctor(s) and my employer. I didn't have a clue as to what to expect tomorrow, next week, or next month. I wanted and needed organized and basic information that would help me get through the moment, the day, and the process.

K.I.S.S. provides guidance from start to finish, through a breast cancer diagnosis and treatments. It offers makeup tips for those days when you look like hell, and answers a plethora of questions: Where did my eyebrows go? How can I wear a bathing suit without boobs? Scarves vs. wigs vs. going bald? What is happening to my toenails? In other words, the important stuff!

K.I.S.S. is organized in sections which, in most cases, will follow the plan of care from the day of diagnosis to the end of treatment (excluding maintenance care), be it three months or your lifetime. At the end of each section, questions are provided to help you know what to ask.

For optimal use of the information provided in this book, it's best to read each section prior to that particular step of treatment.

Why Me? Why Not?

Good and bad things happen throughout our entire lives. When good things happen we never ask, "Why me?" I have never heard anyone say, "Aw, shucks, I just won the lotto...why did it have to be me?" When events are negative, "Why me?" is an understandable question. "Why me?" can represent a range of emotions, including frustration, anger, grief, depression, disgust, fear, anxiety, and self-pity. These are normal reactions to life-altering experiences.

I loathe the expression, "It is what it is." I have always felt it was a cop-out; a way to avoid having to explain something. However, it's the perfect thing to say when the diagnosis is breast cancer. The lifestyles we have chosen and the families we were born into are part of the equation, but they won't guarantee that you will or will not get breast cancer. It really is "what it is."

Acceptance is the key to success. This does not and will not happen overnight. I am five years out from my diagnosis (five years of treatments, surgeries, medications, etc.), and there are days I still have a hard time accepting that I had cancer, let alone the devastation it left behind in my body, mind, and soul. As my acceptance gains strength, "Why me?" loses its power and grip over my life. Remember that you can't tame something you don't acknowledge. Never stop believing in your power, and you will get away from the "whys" and move on to the "hows."

First Things First

This can be a very difficult and stressful time in your life. You are no less of a "good" or "strong" person if you need anti-anxiety or anti-depression medications to help you through this time.

- The medication can help you get through the moment, the day, and the night. It can help you think more clearly and be able to be more proactive in your treatments and recovery. If your physician has not discussed this with you, please talk to her/him. There's no time like the present when it comes to having a clear head and getting a better night's sleep.

- It is wise to have someone with you at each doctor's appointment. Four ears are better than two. It is also a good idea to have paper (note sheets are provided at the end of this book, in the Personal Information Organizer), a pen and/or a tape recorder.

- When someone offers you help, take it! Pride and stubbornness need to take a back seat right now.

- After you have made a final decision about any of the treatments, do not look back.

- You have the final say-so about your treatments, so feel comfortable with your choices.

- Educate yourself a little bit at a time (see the Assistance and Support section for organizational listings).

Activity:

Activity is important and should be addressed in all sections of the book. To keep it simple, we'll touch on it once in First Things First.

When I was diagnosed, someone gave me Lance Armstrong's book *Livestrong*. I read it from cover to cover in about 24 hours, hoping it would give me strength. Instead, I was more anxious by the time I got to the end of the book. I wasn't an athlete, I didn't have his elite medical resources, I wasn't a celebrity, and I looked awful in spandex shorts. Most of us do not have the same physical prowess, ability to focus, or resources that Lance Armstrong has. His book is a wonderful testament of courage and determination; however, it can leave the average Josephine feeling like a failure if she is unable to ride a bike for miles, let alone get out of bed in the morning.

Important:

- **Any activity and exercise is better than none.**
- **Do what you can when you can.**

Exercise Guidelines**

Aerobic Exercise (prolonged, rhythmical exercises that use large muscles)
Note: Do not swim if you are undergoing radiation, have an indwelling catheter or an open wound.
Frequency: 3-5 times per week.
Intensity: "Light" to "moderate." If you cannot hold a conversation, slow down.
Duration: 20-60 minutes. Intermittent bouts are OK.

Resistance/Strength Training (weight or resistance training)
Frequency: 2-3 times per week.
Intensity: 40-60 percent of one maximum repetition ("moderate").
Duration: 1-3 sets of 8-12 repetitions (15 reps maximum).

Flexibility Exercise (stretching or flexibility exercises as shown in the Surgical Section).
Frequency: 2-7 times per week.
Intensity: Slowly reach a point of tension. This should not be painful.
Duration: 4 repetitions of 10-30 seconds per stretch.

- The American College of Sports Medicine's guidelines are in line with the American Cancer Society's recommendations of 30-60 minutes of moderately paced aerobic exercise a minimum of five times per week for cancer survivors.

- **Before starting or continuing with any exercise program, please get clearance from your physician.**

- If unusual symptoms occur, stop exercising and contact your physician.

**American College of Sports Medicine, Guidelines for Exercise Testing and Prescription, Eighth Edition, 2009.

DIAGNOSIS/DEFINITIONS

What is Breast Cancer?

Breast cancer is a malignant (cancerous) growth that begins in the breast. Cancer happens when cells grow in an uncontrolled and abnormal way.

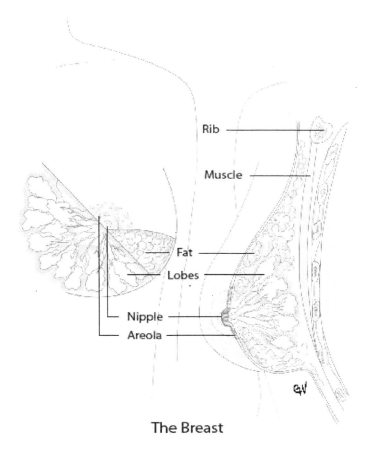

The Breast

Figure 2

What Are the Most Common Types of Breast Cancer?
- Ductal carcinoma (85-90 percent)
- Lobular carcinoma (8 percent)

What Are the Least Common Types of Breast Cancer?
- Inflammatory (skin)
- Paget's (nipple)

Definitions:

Ductal Carcinoma in Situ (DCIS): Cancer which has started in the milk ducts and has not traveled to other tissue.

Inflammatory Breast Cancer (IBC): Cancer which commonly grows in "nests" or "sheets," not lumps. It may look like a rash on the breast. It is not usually detected by a mammogram or ultrasound.

Invasive Ductal Carcinoma (IDC): Cancer which starts in the milk ducts and has invaded the fatty tissue of the breast.

Invasive Lobular Carcinoma (ILC): Cancer which starts in the lobes (base) of the milk ducts. The lobes of the milk ducts are deeper in the breast tissue, which makes it more difficult to detect.

Paget's Disease of the Nipple: Paget's disease of the nipple shows up in and around the nipple. It can present as redness, scaly or flakey skin, a skin irritation, a retraction or dimpling of the nipple, discharge from the nipple, itchiness or tingling. It can look like an orange peel.

Benign: Noncancerous.

Malignant: Cancerous.

Hormone Receptor (estrogen positive or negative): Some breast cancer cells have hormone receptors. These receptors are molecules which allow estrogen and/or progesterone to feed the cells. There are therapies that can help block this action. It is thought that cancers that have positive receptor cells respond well to hormone therapy (HT).

Her2nu Gene: Her2nu-positive tumors tend to grow and spread rapidly. This type of cancer may require aggressive treatment.

Stage of the Cancer: Staging is on a scale of I to IV. The staging is determined by the size of the tumor and how much it has spread. The lower the number, the less extensive the cancer. Additional tissue samples may be needed to determine the stage of the cancer.

BRCA1 and BRCA2: A genetic mutation linked to a higher risk of developing breast, ovarian, colon, and prostate cancers.

Questions to Ask About Your Diagnosis:

- What type of breast cancer do I have?
- What is the size/stage of the tumor?
- Is my tumor estrogen-positive or negative?
- Is my tumor Her2nu-positive or negative?
- What are my treatment options?
- What is your recommendation and why?

TESTS

Tests Used for Diagnosis

Bone Scan: Images of the skeletal system.

Cat Scan (Computer Axial Imaging): Creates 3-D images of the body.

Core Needle Biopsy: A hollow-centered needle is inserted into the lump to remove small samples. Sometimes an ultrasound or X-ray may be used to guide the needle.

Excisional Biopsy: A small cut is made to remove the lump and some surrounding tissue. This is usually an outpatient procedure.

Fine Needle Aspiration: A superfine needle is inserted into the lump and a sample is aspirated (removed by suction).

MRI (Magnetic Resonance Imaging): Radio waves are used to scan tissue. Healthy tissue sends back a different signal than cancerous tissue.

MUGA (Multigated Acquisition Scan): Makes an image of the heart.

PET Scan (Positron Emission Tomography): Produces a digital picture that indicates any changes at a molecular level before they are visible.

Sentinel Node Biopsy (Sentinel – meaning guard or watchdog): The lymphatic system (read more in the section dealing with Lymphedema) drains fluid from your body. The sentinel node is the first node that filters fluid draining away from the area which contains the cancer. Dye is inserted into the tumor, and it will travel to the sentinel node. To see if the cancer has spread, the sentinel node is identified and will be tested for cancer.

TREATMENTS

Treatments

The type, stage, and location of the cancer will direct the recommended treatment options. One or more treatments may be recommended, depending on your specific case.

Surgical:

- **Lumpectomy** is the surgical removal of the part of the breast that contains the cancer (the lump). The surgeon will also take a small amount of the healthy tissue (the margin) which surrounds the tumor.
- **Mastectomy** is the surgical removal of the entire breast.

Radiation:

A treatment that uses high doses of radiation (similar to X-rays) to slow or kill the cancer cells in the area of the tumor.

Chemotherapy (Chemo):

A treatment that uses chemicals to kill cancer cells.

Hormone Therapy:

Some hormones that humans naturally produce help some kinds of cancer grow (estrogen and progesterone). Hormone therapy reduces hormone-receptor-positive cancer cell growth.

Immunotherapy:

Immunotherapy uses the body's immune system to fight certain kinds of cancer.

Getting a Second Opinion

- Many insurance companies cover a second opinion.
- You may need to gather your mammography films, pathology reports/slides, and any blood work you have had done.

- The time it takes to obtain a second opinion should not make your treatment any less effective. Discuss this with your physician.
- It's important that you feel comfortable with your physician and your plan of care.
- If you receive two different recommendations for treatment and feel uncomfortable with having to choose, go for a third opinion.
- Nobody ever regrets getting a second opinion; they only regret not getting one.
- Don't let yourself feel pressured to make an immediate decision. Choosing your treatment plan is an important part of the process and it's OK to take time to think it through.
  - o Many women have recounted how their doctors were on the phone booking surgery three minutes after telling them their diagnosis.
  - o This isn't in your best interest.
  - o Take the time to process the information and discuss it with your family.
- Get a second opinion from a specialist.
  - o If you had a heart problem, wouldn't you go to a heart doctor?
  - o My second opinion was the opposite of the first one I received.

SURGERY

Surgery

Lumpectomy:

The surgical removal of the part of the breast that contains the cancer (the "lump"). They will also take a small amount of healthy tissue (the margin) which surrounds the tumor.

Mastectomy:

The surgical removal of the breast.

- <u>Unilateral</u> (single), meaning removal of one breast.
- <u>Bilateral</u> (double), meaning the removal of both breasts.

Sometimes the physician will recommend removal of the healthy breast as a preventive measure.

Length of Stay in the Hospital (Estimated):

Lumpectomy: Outpatient procedure or overnight.
Mastectomy: One to three days.

** If you want reconstruction, talk to a plastic surgeon about your options prior to undergoing a mastectomy. This way, everyone involved in your care can be coordinated. You may be able to have your reconstruction started at the time of your mastectomy.

A woman who is considering a single mastectomy with implant reconstruction needs to understand that the new breast and the old one will look quite different from each other.

Miscellaneous Topics

Sleeping:

- If it's difficult to get comfortable in bed, try sleeping in a recliner or chair.
- Extra pillows may make you more comfortable in bed.
- You may sleep better in a chair for the first few nights at home.
- Make sure you take your pain medication before going to sleep for the first few nights.

Pain Control:

- It's very important to keep your pain under control for comfort and better healing.
  - If you hurt you won't participate in your recovery, which will slow your recuperation.
- Try to keep your pain level at a "4" or below on a scale of 1-10, "10" being the worst pain in the world
- Don't allow "runaway pain." If pain gets too bad, it will take time to get it back under control. That's time that you could be feeling OK.
- If your medication isn't controlling the pain, contact your physician. Your doctor can't read your mind. You need to let her/him know if the pain medication isn't working.
- Pain medications can cause constipation, so remember to drink lots of water, eat food with fiber, or take an over-the-counter stool softener if this is a problem.

Incisional Care:

- Keep your incision(s) clean.
- Use only soap and water.
- Liquid antibacterial soap is a better choice than bar soap.

- Don't put anything (lotions or creams) on the incision unless instructed by your physician.
- If you have Steri-Strips (thin white tape strips) still on your incisions, do not take them off.
  - o Let them come off on their own.
  - o Pat dry after your shower.

Drains (very important):

- Drains may be needed at the surgical site(s) to get rid of any extra fluid that can accumulate. The drains will be left in for one to four weeks. The number of drains you will have will vary, based on your particular surgery.
- The drain is inserted through a tiny incision and is placed under the skin. A small stitch is used to secure the tubing in place. Be careful not to pull on the tubing.

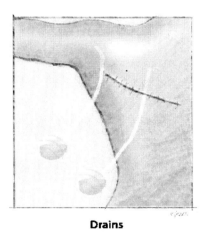

Drains

Figure 3

- You do not want to let the drain/bulb hang loose. The drain should have a soft plastic tab that you can stick a safety pin through, so you can secure it to the inside of your clothing.

- When **showering**, take three to four feet of one-inch inch ribbon and knot the ends together. Place the loop of ribbon around your neck and pin the drains to the ribbon. This will keep the drains from being pulled out when showering. A lanyard for an ID badge works well, too.

- Only take showers. This helps to ensure that any germs are washed away from the incision and down the drain.

- You will be asked to measure the drainage and keep track of it (drainage measuring charts are provided in the Personal Information Organizer section).

- Measuring will be done in units of ml's. Here are some tips to make it easy:

  o Ask your physician for a urine specimen cup to pour your drainage in. The ml's will be noted on the side of the cup and are very easy to read.

  o The bulb at the end of the drain also has ml's noted on the side, but it can be difficult to read.

  o It will be necessary to clear out (strip) the contents of the tubing that leads to the collection bulb at the end of the tubing. Make it easy—use an alcohol wipe to squeeze and slide the contents along the tubing, or wet your thumb and index finger, touch a bar of soap and then squeeze and slide the contents of the tubing into the ball.

- If you wear baggy button-down shirts, the drains easily pin to the inside of the shirt, stay out of the way, and won't be noticed.

  o For convenience, you can make your own "undershirt" with inside pockets to hold the drain(s). This is especially convenient to wear when you go to bed.

    ▪ Sometimes, a hospital will provide you with a camisole to wear that have pockets for the drains. Most insurances cover the first one. They are available in medical supply stores but can be rather expensive.

- Make your own "drain camisole." Take a camisole, tank top, or sleeveless T-shirt and cut it from top to bottom down the front center. Finish the cut edges by folding them over half an inch and stitching them. Add Velcro to make a front closure. Then, on the front lower inside portions, add a pocket for each drain bulb. Estimate the drain bulb to be about the size of a closed fist. Don't worry about what it looks like, because most times you'll be wearing it under clothes or to bed. Its usefulness is more important.

Moving and Stretching with Drains:

- If you have drains in, you will be instructed not to reach above your head until they come out.
- After the drains are removed, it's necessary to do stretching exercises.
- Stretching is covered at the end of this chapter.

What Will I Look Like After Surgery?:

- The first time you look in the mirror after surgery may be difficult.
- Prepare yourself by searching the Internet for "pictures of a mastectomy."
- This is also a good idea for your spouse or significant other to do.

Prosthetics (breast forms):

- These can be ordered at a medical supply company or over the Internet.
- Many insurance companies will cover part or all of the cost.

- You can wear prosthetics in your everyday bra; however, special bras are available. Some insurances will cover mastectomy bras.
- You don't have to spend a lot of money to look "real" under a shirt.
- Prosthetics may range from $30 to $600.
- Lightweight prosthetics are usually more comfortable.
  - o After purchasing some very expensive prosthetics, I wore them once and realized I wasn't a "fake boobs" kind of girl. I donated them to United Way and wondered what the look on someone's face would be when they read the inventory list…"one pair of C-cup boobs."

Incisional Itching:

- Itching may occur at the incision site during the healing process.
- Ask your physician what you can use to calm the itching.

Comfort (if you had lymph nodes removed):

- A small pillow under the affected arm may make it more comfortable.
- In a car, a thin pillow between you and the seat belt may add comfort.
- You may have some numbness/tingling in your chest, under your arm, or in the shoulder area. This may be temporary or permanent.

Shoulder/Arm/Chest Stiffness:

- You may be stiff after surgery.
- Get exercises from your physician or physical therapist. You may also do the stretches shown in this chapter.
- Most patients gain all of their strength and flexibility back in a few months.

Clothing Immediately Following Either Surgery:

- Loose tops that zip or button down the front.
- Comfortable pants.
- Slip-on shoes.

More Thoughts About Tops/Shirts After a Mastectomy:

- If you haven't had reconstructive surgery, clothing can be an emotional issue— especially tops.
- Realistically, most people don't notice or even care if you're "half-chested" or "flat-chested." It took me about four months to realize that.

The following are some tricks that can help you feel better about getting dressed and going out after a mastectomy:

- The use of breast prosthetics (see prosthetics in this section) in a bra is a simple solution. Nobody will know the difference but you.
- Create your own "summer tops" to hold a prosthesis.
  - o Take a halter-style top that has a separated top-to-bottom area (i.e. empire design). It will need to be lined or have two layers of fabric. Make a small slit (about one-half or two-thirds the width of the prosthesis) in the inside fabric, close to the outside edge of the top, and insert the prosthesis. A small snap may be needed to close the opening.

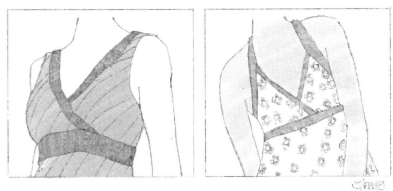

Modifiable Summer Tops

Figure 4

- Look for camisoles and tank tops with built-in bras to hold a prosthesis.

- Halter-style tops look flattering even without prosthetics. The top should not be too loose or too tight in the chest area.

- Dressing in a "layered look" can help camouflage a flat chest.

- Many companies are making bathing suits that look great and have inside pockets for prosthetics (www.landsend.com, www.swimoutlet.com and www.ladyjanebotique.com) or see if your current bathing suit can be modified. You don't have to look like you're wearing your grandmother's bathing suit anymore.

- Lighter-weight prosthetics don't pull fabrics like heavier ones.

- Use your imagination and creativity to modify a variety of different tops. It's easy, inexpensive, and you can still wear them after reconstruction is completed.

Don't Be Afraid to Move After Surgery:

- **You will have a few temporary restrictions (no heavy lifting, no reaching above your head with drains in, and no driving).**

- Don't be afraid to use your arms. You won't damage anything.

- You will feel tightness in the incisional area, but you need to keep your arms moving.

- Using your arm(s) will prevent frozen shoulder, muscle weakness, and reduction in your of range of motion. If you don't use it, you will lose it.

- The more you do your regular daily activities, the faster and better your recovery will be. Just don't overdo it. Doing too much will set you back in your recovery.

Stretching—It's Easy and Necessary

Stretching will help you to:
- Feel good
- Prevent injuries
- Increase relaxation
- Increase circulation
- Increase movement
- Increase normal activities

1. Don't bounce—hold the stretch steady.
2. Don't hold your breath—keep breathing.
3. Feel mild tension—it shouldn't hurt. "Feeling the burn" means you're stretching with too much intensity. Pain is an indicator that something isn't right.
4. Hold each stretch for 10-30 seconds.
5. Do each stretch 4 times, 2-7 times per week.
6. Optimize your "downtime" with stretching.

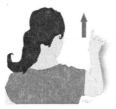

Figure 5

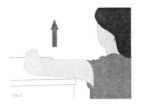

Figure 6

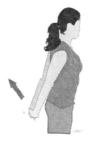

Figure 7

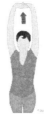

Figure 8

Questions Before Surgery

- What kind of surgery do you recommend and why?
- What other options are available to me?
- Which hospital(s) do you do surgery in?
- How long will I be in the hospital?
- What can I expect during my hospital stay?
- What will I look like after my surgery? Do you have pictures?
- Can reconstruction be started during the initial surgery?
- Can you refer me to a plastic surgeon?
- Will I have a sentinel node biopsy or lymph nodes removed?
- Does a mastectomy reduce my chances of having the cancer return?
  - o   What is the reoccurrence rate?
- Could there be any long-term effects from a lumpectomy?
  - o   What is the reoccurrence rate?
- Will someone instruct me on how to care for my surgical site?
- How long should I expect to be off of work?
- What will my limitations be?
- What are the surgical risks?
- What will be done to control my pain after surgery?
- What can be done to manage any constipation caused by pain medication?
- Are there alternative pain control options?
- How many drains will be inserted?
- Should I have a single or double mastectomy? (If applicable.)

SURGICAL
RECONSTRUCTION

Thoughts About Surgical Reconstruction

Do you really want reconstruction?

- You may feel pressured to make a quick decision about reconstruction—don't! This is something that needs to be thought through, questioned, and discussed.
- Some studies have shown that women who haven't made a snap decision are happier with their choices.
- Radiation treatment and the plastic surgeon's preferences may play into reconstructive decisions.
- Make decisions for the right reasons.
- It's OK to delay your decision regarding reconstruction.
    - Reconstructive surgery can be performed at a later date.
    - It may not bother you to be single- or no-breasted.
        - A model appeared on *Oprah* and indicated that, after her double mastectomy, she chose not to have reconstruction. She said that she felt "cleaner" being flat-chested.
- Reconstruction sounds a lot easier than it really is. It will involve many trips to the plastic surgeon's office, possible complications, additional pain, and more surgeries.
- Stretched skin can itch. Ask your physician if there's anything you can use to help this.
- You can't pick an exact date that your reconstruction will be completed. There are too many variables involved in the process. You will be lucky to guess which season of the year you will be done.

Reconstruction Options:

1. Do nothing.

2. Expanders and implants (most common).

    - This is a **two-step process**.
    - To accommodate implants, you need to expand the skin/muscle with "expanders."
    - Expander(s) will be surgically placed at the time of surgery or at a later date.
    - If you choose the expander and implants:
        o It may be uncomfortable to lie on your stomach.
        o You may feel the implant with certain activities.
        o Your implant may need replacement in the future.
    - Implant surgery has a shorter recovery time than tissue flaps.
    - Expanders and implants require less surgery time.
    - Expanders and implants are less costly.
    - Nipples can be surgically constructed at a later date.
    - The areola (dark area around the nipple) can be tattooed on at a later date.
    - This process isn't like what you see on *Dr. 90210*. It is much more involved.

STEP ONE:

Expanders (picture a sealed, deflated balloon)

- The chest muscle and skin needs to be stretched to make a pocket to hold the implant.
- An expander is surgically placed under the chest muscle.

- At regular intervals (every one to two weeks), you will go to the plastic surgeon's office and she/he will inject the expander with a saline solution to "pump it up."
- This process may take two to six months, depending on a number of circumstances and the "goal size."
- Radiated tissue will respond differently than nonradiated tissue.
- Depending on the plastic surgeon's preference, you will keep the expander in for about one to four months after the last "fill."
- If you have had recent radiation, the plastic surgeon may have you wait six months for the tissue to optimally heal before placement of the expander.
- Filled expanders won't have the same shape as your final implant(s). The expanding tissue may even take on a strange shape. This is temporary.
  - I had one expander mosey into my armpit, and the other looked like an alien was trying to get out through the top. It made for interesting conversation at my stepdaughter's wedding. I had purchased a v-neck dress eight weeks before the wedding and didn't take into account what my expansion could morph into.

STEP TWO:

Implants

- Implants are self-contained pouches that are filled with either saline or silicone and placed under the chest muscle to create a breast mound.
- After expansion is completed, implants are surgically placed.
- Typically, this is an easier surgery than the expander implantation.

- The surgery may be done on an outpatient basis.

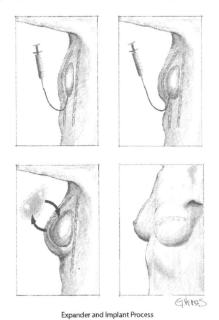

Expander and Implant Process

Figure 9

3. Tram Flap.
   - Tissue from the abdomen is used to make a breast mound.
   - Your hospital stay will be approximately one week.
   - You may have possible long-term abdominal weakness.
   - You automatically receive a tummy tuck using this procedure. If you're thin, you may not have enough tissue for a flap.
   - There is greater post-op discomfort.
   - There are no implants with this surgery.
   - It is an expensive surgery.
   - There is a risk of the flap "not taking hold," requiring further surgeries.

- DIEP Flap is a variation of the tram flap, but only uses skin and fat from the stomach area.

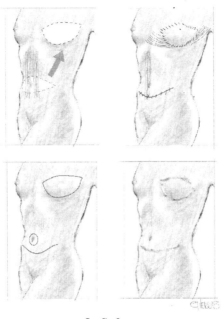

Tram Flap Process

Figure 10

A Note About Nipples

- Nipples can be surgically reconstructed by a plastic surgeon. The doctor may utilize tissue from around the area of the nipple.
- Remember that this is yet another surgery.
  - Areolas (dark area around the nipple):
  - Can be tattooed on.
    - Everyone responds differently to the ink.
    - Ink may or may not fade over time.
    - The tattooing may or may not be painful.
    - The skin may or may not take the ink.

- Radiated tissue may not take the ink the same as unradiated tissue.
  - You can ask for topical lidocaine for the procedure.

Reconstruction Questions

- What kind of reconstructive surgeries are appropriate after my mastectomy?
- Which procedure do you recommend and why?
- What procedure will give me the best results?
- What are the risks?
- What are the benefits?
- How many surgeries will the process require?

Implant-Specific Questions

- What are the risks and benefits of having implants?
- Will I need expanders?
- Do you use saline or silicone implants?
- What are the benefits and risks of each kind of implant?
- Approximately how long do implants last?
- If I have a single implant, how will the look compare to my remaining natural breast?
- How many surgeries are involved in this process?
- How long will the complete process take?
- What will my scars look like?
- Will I have any temporary restrictions?
- How long should I expect to be off of work?
- Will I be able to have nipples made?
- Will I be able to have areolas tattooed?
- Do you have before-and-after pictures?

Tram Flap-Specific Questions

- What are the different tram flap procedures?
- What are the risks and benefits of each procedure?
- How long is the expected recovery period?
- How many surgeries will I need?
- Will insurance cover the surgery?
- Will I have feeling left in my chest/breasts/abdomen?
- Will I be able to have nipples made?
- Will I be able to have areolas tattooed?
- Do you have before-and-after pictures?
- Are there any local plastic surgeons who specialize in this procedure?

CHEMOTHERAPY

Chemotherapy

It's important to remember that everyone responds differently to chemotherapy. One person may experience only partial hair loss, and another may experience everything that chemo offers (that was me).

Consider getting a port inserted prior to your first treatment. A port is a small tube that is inserted into a vein in the chest area for easy access of blood draws and receiving chemo. It won't interfere with your day-to-day activities and can be removed after your treatments are done. It will leave about a one-inch scar.

Helpful Hints on Hair Loss

- Hair thinning or loss may start to happen around the third week of chemotherapy treatment. It will grow back when treatments are done. It may come back a different color or texture.
- Hair may be uncomfortable when falling out.
- You may lose ALL of the hair on your body.
    - I lost all of the hair on my body except on my legs. That's what I call a bad chemo joke.
    - When you go out in public for the first time, you may feel as if everyone "knows" and is staring at you. Trust me, they aren't. People are so focused on what they're doing at the moment, most times they don't notice you— let alone your head. I figured that out when, in a grocery store, a woman almost plowed me over trying to get into the checkout line before me.
    - Many women choose to cut and/or shave their hair before it falls out.
    - **Benefits:**
        - No mess in your shower or on your pillow.

- Lets you be in control of something during an "out of control" situation.
- Shaving is like quickly pulling off a Band-Aid—it's done. It will take your hair a few weeks to completely fall out.
- Make it a family affair. This process can be scary or stressful for some of your immediate family members, too. Let them help you take it off!

- **Children:**
  - If you're concerned about your children's reaction to a "bald mommy," find some pictures on the Internet to show them.
  - Make up a fun and positive story about a bald woman.
  - Let them draw a picture of what they think your new hair will look like when it grows back.
  - Go to a costume shop and get a "scalp cover," and let the kids play with it.

- **Wigs:**
  - You may want to purchase a wig before losing your hair.
  - Wigs come in different sizes. If you can, try it on before you purchase it.
  - Most women who choose to wear a wig don't wear it 100 percent of the time.
  - Check to see if your insurance company will cover all or part of the cost.
  - You may want to wear a skull cap under the wig, as it will help to prevent slipping.
  - Wigs can be hot.
  - Different wigs can give you a new or fun look.

- o Lots of women who experience hair loss prefer a hat, scarf, or going natural (use a wig for special occasions).
- o Be open to changing your preference.
- o Synthetic wigs are less expensive, easier to care for, and look very real.
- o "Look Good…Feel Better" programs will loan wigs at no cost for the duration of your need. For information about a program near you, call (800) 395-LOOK / (800) 395-5665.

- **Scarves (bandanna):**
  - o Buy or make your own to suit your style and needs.
  - o They're easy to care for.
  - o You can find a variety of materials for different occasions and seasons.
  - o Scarves are inexpensive.
  - o Larger scarves vs. the smaller bandanna give you less of the "I'm bald under my scarf" look.
  - o You can purchase "bangs of hair" to place under the forehead of your scarf. The look is very real.

- **Storing Your Scarves:**
  - o Take about four feet of cloth/ribbon (two to three inches wide), poke a hole about two inches from the end, and hang the strip on a hook attached to your bathroom door, closet, etc. Use clothespins to clip each scarf onto the strip. This will help keep them organized and clean.

Skin Care

- Moisturize, moisturize, moisturize!
- Stay hydrated by drinking lots of water and other fluids.

Makeup

- A little bit can go a long way to making you feel "more normal."
- "Look Good...Feel Better," (800) 395-LOOK, can help with free makeup and advice.
- You will need to adjust your makeup routine.
- Be careful with bold colors; they may make you look more washed out.
- Eyebrow kits are now available on the Internet and in most drug stores. They usually provide a brush, powder, and stencil to help create the perfect eyebrow.
- Try false eyelashes. They work and are inexpensive.

Going to Treatment

- Have a driver for your treatments. If you're in need, the American Cancer Society may be able to provide assistance (see Assistance and Support section).

Immune System Protection

- Wash your hands regularly.
- If possible, avoid being around people who are sick.
- Avoid crowds.
- Avoid buffet-style restaurants.
- You don't have to be housebound— just be sure to take precautions.
- Ask your physician about a flu/pneumonia shot.

Insomnia

- Insomnia is common during chemo because of steroids you receive during treatment.
- Speak to your physician about getting a sleep aid.

- If the prescribed dose doesn't work, speak to your physician again.
- Be persistent—sleeplessness doesn't have to be an issue.
- A good sleep will make a big difference in healing, outlook, and attitude.
  - My insomnia was awful. I spent many nights watching infomercials or religious programs because that was all that was on at 2 a.m. on our local cable. The running joke was that I had to keep the credit cards put away because at that hour, when you're bored and exhausted, ordering a collapsible ladder, a forest-green suede vest (with fringe), or enough makeup for a year sounds like a marvelous idea. I don't wear vests or makeup, and my husband needs another ladder like a hole in the head.

Clothing

- A female comedian was at her lowest when she tried to make a joke out of "What's with women going through chemo and wearing sweat suits out in public?" Shame on her! Comfortable is what you will want to be and, really, who cares what someone else thinks?

Windows of Opportunity (moments of feeling good)

- When you feel good, take advantage of it.
- Don't try to be "Wonder Woman" when you're feeling good.

Teeth

- If possible, get your teeth cleaned before treatment starts. Germs are released during a cleaning.

Sores in the Mouth (this is a possibility)

- Stay on top of it!

- Homemade mouth rinse:
  - o 1 cup warm water
  - o 1/4 teaspoon baking soda
  - o 1/8 teaspoon salt
- Rinse with solution, and then rinse with plain water.
- Keep the solution next to your sink and use it three times a day.

Vitamins

- Ask your physician if any of your supplements may interfere with the effectiveness of the chemotherapy or if there's anything you need to take to boost your immunity.

Constipation

- Constipation is very common during chemotherapy.
- Constipation can be debilitating and painful, and can cause hemorrhoids.
- Try prune juice daily.
- Try senna tea from the health food store.
- Over-the-counter stool softeners and milk of magnesia may help constipation.
- "The Blaster":
  - o Mix 1/4 cup of prune juice and one recommended dose of milk of magnesia, and warm it in the microwave.
- Eat a quality variety of yogurt.
- Eat high-fiber foods.
- Thirty minutes of moderate exercise can help constipation.
- Drink plenty of water.

Food

- A healthy and balanced diet is the best course of action, but not always possible.

- Be careful of spicy foods.
- Consider nutritional supplements if eating is difficult. You can try Boost, Ensure, Carnation Instant Breakfast, etc.
- Ginger ale, Popsicles, and soup are good to have around.
- Don't eat your favorite foods at this time because, if there is a change in your taste buds, you may dislike these foods when things get back to normal.
  - I can never eat another turkey roll-up from the cafeteria at work. I would always buy one to take with me for lunch during my treatments.
- BUT, any food is better than none.
- You may find you get strange food cravings. This is normal.
  - I craved McDonald's French fries and cinnamon-coated Pop-Tarts for about six consecutive days at one point.

Smells

- Some smells may become bothersome. This will improve after chemo is finished.
- Breathe through your mouth if smells bother you.

Nausea

- If you're bothered by nausea, the following may help:
  - Ginger ale
  - Physician-prescribed medications.
  - Tiny spoonfuls of quality yogurt.
  - The scent of peppermint can help soothe an upset stomach (oil, candy, or tea).
  - Place a few fresh slices of ginger root in a cup of boiling water. Let it cool before drinking.
  - Popsicles or flavored ice cubes.

    o Cold and room-temperature foods can help reduce nausea.

    o Pinch your "anti-nausea" point. This is located on the muscles between your thumb and first finger. Try several locations until you find the "tender spot."

Neuropathy (nerve damage)

- Neuropathy can cause discomfort or pain.
- The most common places to be affected are the hands, feet, and legs.
- If neuropathy becomes an issue, there are medications that help. Call your physician.

Temporary Memory Loss

- This is also called "chemo brain."
- Write reminders on Post-it notes or in a notebook.
- Use a Dictaphone.
- People will try to convince you that your memory loss is due to the situation or that it's because you're getting older...blah, blah, blah.

Weight Gain

- This isn't the time to worry about your weight.
- It's common to gain 20-40 pounds (OMG).
- Any exercise or activity is better than none. So don't beat yourself up if your exercise for the day consists of getting out of bed and diving onto the couch.

Cuticles

- Can get very dry.
- Moisturize hands and cuticles daily.
- Don't cut cuticles. Gently push them back when they're damp.

Fingernails

- Fingernails and toenails are made from the same materials as hair.
- Nails can become brittle, discolored and, on rare occasions, they may lift and fall off.
- This isn't the time to be getting artificial nails.
- Keep your nails short and filed.

Menopause

- Menopause can be induced by chemotherapy or hormone receptor medications.
- This can be temporary, permanent, or partial.
- If you have hot flashes:
  o Soy and flaxseed products have been shown to help relieve hot flashes (check with your oncologist before eating soy products).
  o Flaxseed can be ground and added into foods such as salads, or mixed into shakes. Start with small amounts.
  o Moderate aerobic exercise may help.
  o Your physician may prescribe medications that can ease symptoms.
  o Drink six to eight glasses of water a day.
  o Avoid sugar and refined/processed foods.
  o Avoid caffeine.
  o Maintain an ideal body weight.

Pain Control

- If you don't tell your physician about any pain, he/she won't know about it.
- Ask what can be done to control your pain.

Accepting Help

- This isn't the time to be "Wonder Woman." If people want to help, **ACCEPT IT!** My husband is laughing as I write this part. I was pretty independent (he says stubborn) prior to my diagnosis, and it was difficult for me to say "OK, help away," or to at least let someone do something for me. This is a way for friends and family to show their support during your treatments.

Getting Out of the House

- Get out of the house when appropriate. Normal routines will be upset by chemo, so when the opportunity arises to do something out of the house, go for it.
  - o I would go out whenever I had my "window of opportunity." I knew I had about two hours until I pooped out and had to go home. One day when I was out, my feet swelled up so bad that it hurt too much to have shoes on. I was determined not to waste time by heading home. I picked up a pair of slippers in the store I happed to be in, threw them on at the register, finished my shopping, and then went next door to quiet my carbohydrate cravings. So there I sat in a restaurant, wearing slippers, with a bald head and two big plates in front of me loaded with mashed potatoes, pizza, macaroni and cheese, French fries, and cake.

Emotions

- Emotions can be a roller-coaster ride during your chemo. If need be, please consult your physician regarding medication to help.
- You aren't less of a person if you ask for antidepressants.
- Seek out a local support group to help you during chemo.
- See the section on Coping for more information.

Flatulence

- "Chemo farts" have a life all their own. Need I say more?

Noise

- Some women experience a temporary sensitivity to noises. This is normal. You may need quiet. Or, like me, you might need to have the television on low all the time. I used to joke that the TV was my babysitter.

Medical Marijuana

- Medical literature indicates that medical marijuana can help relieve nausea, vomiting, reduction of appetite, and unintentional weight loss. As of this book's publication date, there are 13 states in the U.S. that have legalized the use of medical marijuana when prescribed by a physician.

"Feelings" When Chemo is Completed

- After you're finished with your last treatment, it's common to experience a feeling of being alone, being anxious, or being scared. You may feel like you're not "fighting the fight" anymore, or have lost your "back-up." This will pass. The chemo has done its job!

Medications

- Your bathroom counter will fill up with medications. Get a small, flat-bottomed basket to keep them organized and in one location.

Irregular Heartbeats

- If you experience irregular heartbeats, contact your physician.

Bonus!

- Many women notice that after chemo is completed, they have a clearer complexion and less acne.

Chemotherapy Questions

- Why do I need chemotherapy?
- What drugs will be used and why?
- What could happen if I don't have chemo?
- How often will I receive treatments?
- How many weeks/months will the treatments last?
- Where will I have the treatments done?
- How will the chemo be given?
- Should I get a port-a-cath?
- What are some of the side effects and how long will they last?
- What are the risks of chemo?
- Can I get a flu shot while receiving chemo?
- Can I work during chemo?
- Will I receive anti-nausea medications?
- How successful is the treatment for my type of cancer?
- Do I need to stay away from sick people?
- Can I exercise?
- Can I eat before my treatments?
- Can I take vitamins?

Clinical Trials

- What is a clinical trial?
    - A chemotherapy clinical trial is a study of the drugs, conducted for effectiveness, using no less than the current standard of medical care.
    - Participation is voluntary.

Questions to Ask About Clinical Trials

- What are the benefits of participating in a clinical trial?
- Are there any risks in participating in a clinical trial?
- Can I drop out of a clinical trial at any time?

RADIATION

Radiation

Radiation treatment uses high doses of radiation (similar to X-rays), directed in a beam, to slow or kill cancer cells in the area of the tumor.

- Everyone's skin responds differently to radiation treatment.
  - o You may get anything from a light suntan up to burns in the radiated area.
- They will need to do a "mapping" of the area prior to starting treatment.
  - o This is a one-time process.
  - o It takes about 30-40 minutes.
  - o You will need to remain very still and in the same position during this time. Ask your physician for something to relax you if you believe you may have a difficult time remaining still.
- Treatments do not hurt.
  - o Treatments are usually in a series of 20-30 visits (Monday through Friday for five to seven weeks).
  - o Schedule this into your daily routine.
  - o Total time per treatment is about 20 minutes.
  - o You will be told to have no creams or lotions on your skin during treatment.
- You will be required to put on a gown when you go in for treatment. For ease of changing, wear a button or zip-down top and leave your bra at home, if possible.
- If the radiated area becomes uncomfortable, **do not** place cold or hot packs on it. Lukewarm compresses are best.
  - o Radiated tissue may become itchy. DO NOT scratch this area.
  - o Fatigue can become an issue.
  - o Do what you can when you can.
  - o Be easy on yourself.

- Accept help from others.
  - ○ Save your energy for what you want to do.
  - ○ Reduce stress by keeping a lighter schedule.
- Fatigue may last for a few months after your last treatment.
- Watch out for sunburn on your radiated area during and after treatments.
  - ○ Protect the radiated area for up to six months after your last treatment.
  - ○ Use sunscreen (if you don't have open sores) that's SPF 30 or greater.
- Physicians recommend only water-based products on the radiated areas. Pure aloe is best.
- You may get radiation burns. If this occurs, keep the area clean. If it becomes uncomfortable, you can use Domeboro astringent solution for skin irritation.
  - ○ If the burn oozes, you can place nonstick gauze over the area to prevent it from sticking to your shirt. Don't place tape on the affected area.

Skin Care

- Stay hydrated.
- You can use pure aloe on the radiated area only **after** daily treatment is completed.

Burns

- Keep the area clean.
- You can use pure aloe after treatments.
- Use nonstick gauze to help prevent any oozing sores from sticking to your shirt.
- Use paper tape outside of the affected area to hold gauze in place.

- Glad Press'n Seal is another option to help hold gauze in place. Cut it into strips and be sure not to place it on the treated area.
- A warm compress of Domeboro can help with healing. This can be found in any drug store.
- Watch for signs of infection and contact your physician if they're present.

Vitamins

- Ask your physician if your supplements may interfere with the effectiveness of the radiation.

Itching

- Topical prescriptions from your physician are available.
- Pressure on the radiated area can help alleviate itching. Sleep on your stomach or use a pillow.
- Eat an apple a day, as pectin in the apple may help with healing.
- Wear soft clothing.
- Do not scratch, rub, or scrub the treated area. This can lead to infection.

Radiation Questions

- Why do I need radiation?
- What does "mapping" mean?
- Will you give me an anti-anxiety medication prior to mapping?
- Why is mapping needed?
- Will I have any restrictions?
- Do I need to limit my regular activities?
- Do I need to stay out of the sun?
- Do I need to stay away from sick people?
- Can I exercise?
- Can I have reconstructive surgery if I have radiation?
- Do the benefits of radiation continue after treatment stops?
- Can I have radiation without other treatments?
- Will any side effects be temporary or permanent?
- What happens if I need to miss a few treatments?
- What are my chances of the cancer recurring and/or spreading if I don't have radiation?
- How do I know if the treatments are working?
- What side effects of radiation need to be reported ASAP?
- How many sessions are recommended?

HORMONE THERAPY/
IMMUNOTHERAPY

Hormone Therapy

What is Hormone Therapy?

- Some breast cancers grow because they're sensitive to estrogen and/or progesterone ("estrogen and/or progesterone-receptor positive") (ER+/PR+).
- A test will be done to see if you are estrogen receptor negative or positive.
- If your tumor is "estrogen and/or progesterone-receptor positive," you may be offered hormone therapy.
- **Hormone therapy is the opposite of hormone replacement therapy.**
- Hormone therapy is a medication that can help slow cancer cell growth or stop cancer cells from multiplying.
- Hormone therapy may affect bone density.
    - o This may require an annual bone density test.
    - o Preventive measures can be taken to protect your bones, so to speak, with your oncologist.

Hormone Therapy Questions

- Is my cancer estrogen-receptor or progesterone-receptor positive or negative?
- Do I need hormone therapy?
- What will hormone therapy do?
- Which one do you recommend?
- How long will I be taking this drug?
- Are there any side effects I might expect?
- Are there risks involved?
- What might happen if I choose not to do hormone therapy?
- How long will I need to take hormone therapy?

- How will hormone therapy affect my chances of having children?
- Will hormone therapy affect my ability to have sex?
- Are you aware of any financial assistance available for the medication?
- Will my insurance cover this?

What is Immunotherapy?

- Some breast cancers begin when a gene called Her2nu becomes confused and makes cells divide and grow, turning into cancer.
- An intravenous (IV) drug (Herceptin) can be given to help slow or stop the Her2nu-positive cancer cells.

Immunotherapy Questions:

- Is my cancer Her2nu positive or negative?
- Do I need treatment?
- How often will I receive treatment?
- How many treatments will I need?
- Can this be done with a port?
- Are there risks involved?
- Are there any side effects I might expect?
- Do you provide the treatment in your office?
- Will my insurance cover this?

LYMPHEDEMA

Lymphedema

What is Lymphedema?

- Lymphedema occurs when lymphatic fluid builds up in soft tissue.
- Lymphatic fluid is part of the immune system that helps fight illness, and is made of proteins, fat, and red and white blood cells.
- Lymphedema can cause pain and swelling.
- Lymphedema can occur following the removal of even one lymph node.

If you have had **any** lymph nodes removed, the prevention of lymphedema should become part of your daily life.

The following preventive tips are directed at the affected limb:

- Avoid needle sticks (shots and blood draws) from the affected limb.
- Avoid cutting cuticles—push them back instead.
- Moisturize your arm. Start at your fingers, applying in only one direction, and gently work your way to your shoulder.
- Avoid extremely hot showers.
- Wear gloves when doing dishes.
- Avoid saunas, hot tubs, and steam baths.
- Avoid tight-fitting jewelry.
- Avoid tight and restrictive clothing.
- Prevent sunburns by using a 30 SPF or greater sunscreen.
- Only have a therapeutic lymphedema massage by a **certified professional**.
- Wear gloves when gardening.
- Avoid carrying heavy objects, especially when your arm is extended down.

- Carry your purse on the "other shoulder."
- Wear your bra a little looser rather than tighter.
- Avoid taking your blood pressure on the affected side. If both breasts were involved, the blood pressure reading can be taken on your leg.
- Don't smoke.
- Avoid alcohol and caffeine.
- Monitor your salt intake.
- Avoid heating pads or heat treatments to the entire area (neck, back, shoulder, chest, and arm).
- Avoid deep-tissue massage on the affected area.
- Use caution when using a razor to shave under your arms. An electric razor is preferable.
- Use caution and oven mitts when handling hot objects.
- Immediately wash all cuts/scrapes with soap and water.
- Apply antibiotic cream to cuts and scrapes (if you don't have an allergy to it), and cover the area.
- Use insect repellant to avoid bug bites.
- Wear a compression sleeve when flying.
  - A compression sleeve is like support hose made for the arm.
  - Compression sleeves are skin-colored.
- If you have diabetes, carefully manage your blood glucose.
- Elevate your arm when at rest (when possible).
- Do not overtax your arm with activity or exercise.
- If your arm feels tired or achy, it's time for a break.

Do not ignore these signs and symptoms of lymphedema

- Signs of infection
  - Fever

- o Redness
- o Swelling
- o Warm to the touch
- Signs of lymphedema
  - o Feeling of heaviness in the arm
  - o New onset of skin sensitivity
  - o Loss of feeling
  - o Redness
  - o Weeping or oozing rashes
  - o Itching
  - o Pain/throbbing

Keep a compression sleeve or Ace bandage handy. Your insurance company may cover the cost of a sleeve.

Most physical therapists and massage therapists have had little instruction about lymphedma during their training. When dealing with lymphedema issues, you want a **certified professional**. Check your local hospitals and clinics.

COPING

Coping

You may feel that you have lost control of your body. Remember that you haven't lost control of your life. Take the time to recognize what you can control and who you can count on.

There is no magic formula to get through this storm. Everyone is different when it comes to coping skills. There is no right or wrong way to cope.

- A wise woman asks how, not why.
- Fear, anger, and feelings of "loss" are common and normal. Don't be afraid to recognize any emotions.
- You may need to start a dialogue with some people.
    o   They may be afraid of making you feel worse.
    o   They may be afraid of the situation.
    o   They may not know what to say.
- Laugh, sing, scream, and cry. These all help strengthen the immune system and feel good, too!
- Try not to shut friends and family out.
- Watch funny movies.
- Pray, keep your faith.
- Keep a journal.
- Keep up with exercise and activities, as tolerated.
- Allow yourself to do "nothing"—it's all about you!
- Practice positive imagery.
- Accept what others have to offer.
- Try relaxation, yoga, meditation, and deep breathing.
- Attend support groups.
- Don't look too far ahead. Smaller time frames are easier to grasp when dealing with surgeries and treatments.

- "Post-treatment blues" are normal, but not mandatory. They can last weeks or even months. If they continue too long, seek professional help.

- Don't look back on any of your decisions or actions. You can't change the past.

- Even though this may be a difficult time, remember it's OK to laugh and have fun.

- Take one day at a time.

- Things aren't black and white.

- Good always comes out of bad. You may see it today, tomorrow, next week, or not until next year...but it will be there, waiting for you.

People will say dumb things. Get used to it. Usually, it isn't intentional. People don't always know what to say, or they're afraid to say anything, thinking they will make you feel bad. They may be nervous or just idiots. No matter, give them the benefit of the doubt.

- A patient I was working with asked me, "What the hell did you do to your hair?" I wanted to say, "Right back at ya, buddy." He had less hair than I did.

- I had another patient tell me they liked my pirate costume. It was Halloween, and I had on a scarf that matched my scrubs. All I could muster was a "thank you."

- A waitress made a sarcastic remark about my bald head, thinking I was trying to make a fashion statement.

- Prior to my double mastectomy, a co-worker told me it was no big deal to lose my boobs, since "boobs don't make the woman." I understood what he meant, but it sure came out the wrong way.

People will want to tell you about somebody who knows somebody who went through this, or how their great Aunt Olive died from breast cancer nine years ago. If you aren't comfortable with any conversation, it's OK to say, "I'd rather not talk about this right now."

Sweet Snippet:

When a friend of mine would go to the doctor's, and knowing she would be weighed, she would put her prosthesis in her purse before she would step on the scale. Only a real woman would understand that!

A New Normal

As each day passes, you will be developing a "new normal." You may not see it at the time, but one day you will say "aha." Embrace each new part of your life.

- Different perspectives
- Different pace of daily activities
- Different priorities
- Different needs
- Different relationships
- Different empathies
- Different tolerance/patience levels

I Had to Bite My Tongue so I Wouldn't Laugh:

I work in a hospital with people who have just had open-heart surgery. On rare occasions, and if the situation is appropriate, I will relate part of my story (double mastectomy with six surgeries on my chest). My goal is for them to feel that they aren't alone and they will make it through recovery. I told a patient my story and later, when his family came in for a visit, I happened to be in the room. He introduced me to his family, and proceeded to tell them that I had had a breast reduction. Oh, my.

FAMILY AND CHILDREN

Family and Children

- Whatever you're feeling, your family is feeling it too.
- Your family wants to help, but may feel helpless. Let them be involved. Of course, keep age-appropriateness of the children in mind.
- Communicate, communicate, and then communicate some more.
- Evil likes to divide and conquer. At this time, relationships can be broken apart if there is an existing fracture. On the other hand, some relationships become stronger because people pull together for a cause and let the "small things" go.
- Children mimic the reactions and attitudes of adults. Keep it positive but realistic.
- Accept your family's help and support. It is OK and even necessary, at times, to ask for it.
- Knowledge is power! Educate yourself.
- Ask your children what they're feeling. Let them know it's OK to feel whatever it is they're feeling.
- Let children know they can't "catch mommy's illness" like a cold.
- Keep children informed as to what the next step is and what to expect.
- Use a calendar to mark significant dates and let the children cross them off. For example: Cross off each radiation treatment or each doctor's visit.
- Encourage siblings to help each other.
- Let the children make choices and do more chores, such as folding clothes, washing dishes, sweeping, and walking the dog. Tell them it doesn't need to be perfect; you just

appreciate their help. They will grow from helping with these responsibilities.

- Children may become distracted during this time. Encourage them to express themselves by writing, drawing, or even talking to their friends or a trusted adult.

- Don't forget that kids still need to be kids and do "kid stuff."

- Don't underestimate a child's insight. Keep things simple and straightforward.

- Don't forget about informing estranged children or family members. This could lead to improved family dynamics.

- Humor with children can be a wonderful communication tool. You can say things like: "I'm going to be bald like Humpty Dumpty," or, "Mommy's medicine may make her throw up, like Fido does when he eats garbage."

Kids' Snippets:

- One Christmas, a woman let her small children decorate the tree all by themselves. The tree stood so proud and mighty in the living room when the children were done. They were so happy that they had done it all by themselves for their mom, and nobody cared that only the bottom fourth of the tree was decorated.

- A woman had her 6- and 8-year-old grandsons for Halloween. She was at her wit's end as to what to do, since she had thought her daughter would have been feeling better when the date rolled around. So they all played dress-up with her husband's clothes, and all three of them went trick-or-treating as "grandpa."

ASSISTANCE AND SUPPORT

Assistance and Support

Contact the American Cancer Society at www.cancer.org
Possible financial assistance for medical needs.

- Possible transportation during treatments.
- Education.
- *TLC,* a magazine and catalog that offers a wide variety of wigs, hats, prosthetics, swimwear, and additional accessories at low prices.

Other Resources:

BREASTCANCER.ORG, www.breastcancer.org

Breast Cancer Society of Canada, www.bcsc.ca; (800) 567-8767

Cancer Care Inc., www.cancercare.org; (800) 813-4673

Centers for Disease Control and Prevention, www.cdc.gov; (800) 232-4636

Department of Veterans Affairs, www.va.gov; for local offices, call (800) 827-1000

Living Beyond Breast Cancer, www.lbbc.org; (888) 753-5222

Look Good...Feel Better, www.lookgoodfeelbetter.org

National Cancer Institute, www.nci.nih.gov; (800) 422-6237

National Lymphedema Network, www.lymphnet.org; (800) 541-3259

Social Security Administration, www.ssa.gov; (800) 772-1213

The Susan G. Komen Foundation, ww5.komen.org; (877) 465-6636

Cure magazine (free), www.curetoday.com

MD Anderson Cancer Center, www.mdanderson.org

Family Medical Leave Act (FMLA), www.dol.gov/ESA/WHD/FMLA

Health Care Financing Administration (HCFA), www.cms.hhs.gov; (800) 447-8477

Pharmaceutical Assistance, www.needymeds.org

Cancer Financial Assistance Coalition, www.cancerfac.org/reading/sources.php

WORK-RELATED
QUESTIONS

Work-Related Questions

- What is FMLA (Family Medical Leave Act)?
- What is STD (Short Term Disability)?
- What is the difference between FMLA and STD?
- Am I eligible for STD?
- How is my company's STD structured?
- How does my STD paperwork need to be written?
- Can I connect multiple surgeries/treatments on one leave?
- What is intermittent STD?
- Can employees donate sick time?

PERSONAL
INFORMATION
ORGANIZER

Information Organizer

Name: _____

Address: _____

_____

Home Phone: _____

Cell: _____

Office: _____

Emergency Contact: _____

Phone: _____

Allergies: _____

Insurance Information

Company: _____

Subscriber: _____

Contract: _____

Plan: _____

Group: _____

Phone: _____

Company: _____

Subscriber: _____

Contract: _____

Plan: _____

Group: _____

Phone:

Misc. _____

_____

Physicians

Family Physician
Name: _____
Address: _____

_____
Phone: _____
Fax: _____

Oncologist
Name: _____
Address: _____

_____
Phone: _____
Fax: _____

Surgeon
Name: _____
Address: _____

_____
Phone: _____
Fax: _____

Radiologist
Name: _____
Address: _____

_____
Phone: _____
Fax: _____

Other
Name: _____
Address: _____

_____
Phone: _____
Fax: _____

Pharmacy

Name: _____

Phone: _____

Fax: _____

Medications

Medication	Dose	Times-A-Day

Notes

Notes

Notes

Notes

DRAINAGE OUTPUT CHART

Day	A.M.	Noon	P.M.	Totals
1				
2				
3				
4				
5				
6				
7				
8				
9				
10				
11				
12				
13				
14				
15				
16				
17				
18				
19				
20				
21				
22				
23				
24				
25				
26				
27				
28				
29				
30				
31				

DRAINAGE OUTPUT CHART

Day	A.M.	Noon	P.M.	Totals
1				
2				
3				
4				
5				
6				
7				
8				
9				
10				
11				
12				
13				
14				
15				
16				
17				
18				
19				
20				
21				
22				
23				
24				
25				
26				
27				
28				
29				
30				
31				

DRAINAGE OUTPUT CHART

Day	A.M.	Noon	P.M.	Totals
1				
2				
3				
4				
5				
6				
7				
8				
9				
10				
11				
12				
13				
14				
15				
16				
17				
18				
19				
20				
21				
22				
23				
24				
25				
26				
27				
28				
29				
30				
31				

DRAINAGE OUTPUT CHART

Day	A.M.	Noon	P.M.	Totals
1				
2				
3				
4				
5				
6				
7				
8				
9				
10				
11				
12				
13				
14				
15				
16				
17				
18				
19				
20				
21				
22				
23				
24				
25				
26				
27				
28				
29				
30				
31				